Detox:

Natural Recipes to Cleanse, Rejuvenate, Recharge & Renew your Body

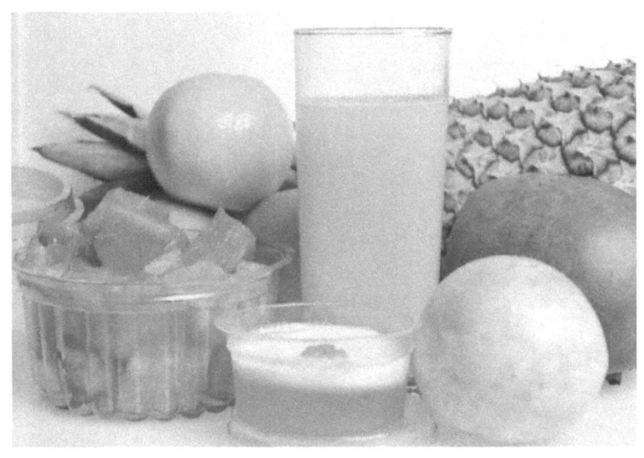

By Bandana Ojha

All rights Reserved ©2020

Chapters:

Introduction

Detoxification is a process by which the body gets rid of unwanted toxins which are acquired because of environmental pollutants, chemicals, pesticides, excessive consumption of junk, refined and processed foods. A well-designed cleanse enhances the functions of the detoxification organs and helps us regain balance. If you have any problem like dry skin, skin rashes, hair loss, fatigue, lethargic feeling, drowsiness, tiredness, body pain, problem sleeping , excessive body weight, swollen joints, stiff neck, cramps, abdominal or lower back pain then a full body cleanse could help you to get the solution of all your problems. This book is the ultimate guide to cleanse and detox all the toxins out of your body. Discover a more vibrant, glowing, healthy and full-of-life going through this book and cleanse, rejuvenate, recharge, renew your body with simple recipes with ingredients which are available in your kitchen.

Kidney Detox

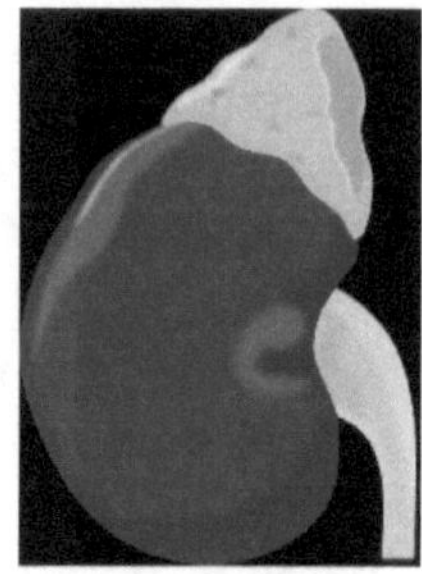

Ten signs your kidney is telling you, it needs help:

dry skin, skin rashes, hair loss

fatigue, lethargic feeling, drowsiness

heart palpitations, high blood pressure

incontinence, kidney stones, urinary tract infections

decreased urine flow increased nightly urination

burning or painful urination, dark colored urine

itching, sleep problems, metallic taste in mouth

nausea, coldness, fever

swollen joints, stiff neck, cramps

abdominal or lower back pain

poor appetite, diabetes, anemia

Foods That Are Bad for Your Kidneys

Dairy

The kidneys need to maintain a proper balance of the calcium and phosphorous minerals, removing away the excess under normal circumstances. With kidney disease, the kidneys don't filter away the excess like they should, making dairy less safe to consume. Instead of removing the extra phosphorous, the kidneys will grab calcium from the bones to help keep the balance together. It helps to limit phosphorous-heavy foods with kidney disease, such as yogurt, cheese and milk, to help keep the balance closer to normal levels.

Meat

While consuming meat in general isn't particularly harmful, having too much of it in your diet isn't good for your kidneys. Excess protein in your diet can create or exacerbate existing renal issues because of the burden protein places on the kidneys. With the extra weight wearing on the kidneys, it's harder to remove urea waste from the body. In fact, excess meat can also cause calcium oxalate stones to form due to the acidic residue animal meat leaves behind. The body favors an alkaline state, so it tries to remove calcium to return to it. Not only will your bones suffer for it, but the stones don't feel good either.

Artificial Sweeteners

It's easy to want to consume an artificial sweetener instead of regular sugar; after all, sugar does little for the body other than add calories, and sweeteners are don't cost any in your day. While this might be true for a more natural sweetener like Stevia, artificial ones like Splenda or aspartame can harm the body. When consuming two diet sodas a day, there is a greater risk for developing kidney disease or similar problems with the renal system. Neither artificial sweeteners nor sugar are the better alternative; stick with fruits or a dab or Stevia if a sweet tooth really strikes.

Caffeine

Although not precisely a food in the true sense of the word, but enough people drink coffee and treat it as a meal for it to count. It's extremely easy to become dependent on caffeine, even needing it in the middle of the day for a burst after the morning dose wears off. However, as a strong stimulant, it has a potentially profound effect on the kidneys. Those who already have worn kidneys are more likely to develop problems with long-term caffeine use. Drinking caffeine increases the rate at which calcium is extracted from the body and makes the user more likely to develop kidney stones later.

Excess Painkillers

Another consumable that can negatively affect the kidneys excess painkillers, especially when taking high amounts over a long period of time. One of the worst culprits are nonsteroidal anti-inflammatory drugs, or NSAIDs. As many as 3 percent of chronic kidney diseases each year are believed to be due to taking too many NSAIDs like ibuprofen. Over-the-counter and prescription medications are both potentially harmful to the kidneys when taken in excess. Never take more than the packaging or your doctor prescribes; when in doubt, speak with your physician about any specific problems you're having and what kind of alternatives may be available for treatment.

Smoking

Tobacco is a harmful substance that offers no health benefits for its users. The ramifications of smoking cigarettes even once or around non-smokers are well-known, but you may not know that it's directly dangerous to the kidneys as well. Smokers are more likely to urinate excess protein. In addition, diseases that cause kidney problems like diabetes and hypertension are only made much worse by smoking cigarettes. In fact, smokers are more likely to have worse kidneys that fail and are more likely to require dialysis as a result

Foods and herbs that may keep the kidneys clean

Those who wonder how to detox kidneys naturally are often surprised to learn that there are many delicious foods and herbs that can help. For instance, kidney cleansing with herbs can involve a variety of options. In terms of foods that are good for kidney cleansing, nutrient-dense, high antioxidant choices are best. Foods high in electrolytes are good for cleansing, too. These are the list of food items that are good kidney cleanse options.

Cranberries, Black cherries, Blueberries, Watermelon, Beets, Spinach, Seaweed, Lemon juice, Asparagus, Ginger, Barley, Millet, Pumpkin seeds ,Spirulina, Grapes

**Detox drinks to cleanse kidneys**

Watermelon Juice for a nice Kidney Cleanse:

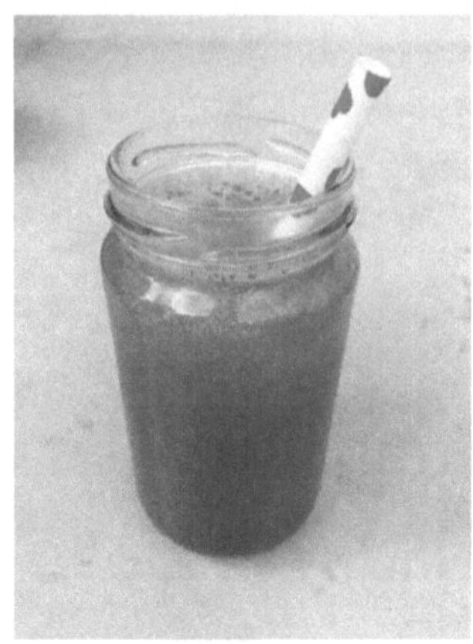

Watermelon is an amazing source of potassium and is also rich with water (99%). So, this would wonderfully help you in flushing out the toxins from your body. Here is the juice recipe of watermelon to cleanse kidneys.

Things You Need:
Watermelon Slices- 2-3 cups
Peeled Lime -1
Honey- ¼ tsp

Things You Should Do:
Blend the watermelon slices and peeled lime together.
Add honey to it and stir them well.
Now, drink this delicious juice to clean your kidneys.

Beet Juice to Clean Kidneys:

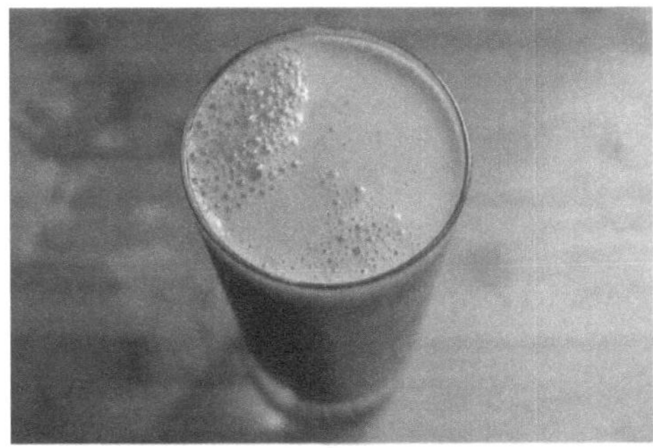

Beets are extremely healthy. It is well equipped with antioxidants and can extravagantly increase the acid content of urine.

Things You Need:
Large Peeled Beet- 1
Fresh Peeled Ginger- 1
Ice cubes- 2-3
Things You Should Do:
Blend the above-mentioned ingredients thoroughly.
Serve fresh with ice cubes.
Drink this juice regularly to clean your kidneys.

Lemon Juice for kidney cleansing:

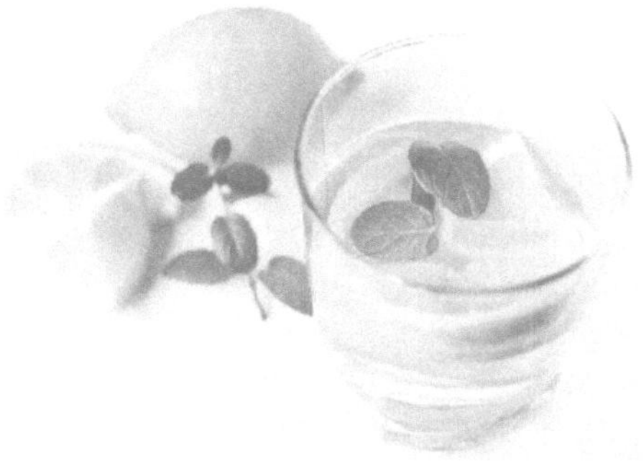

Lemon Juice contains Vitamin C and Citric acid, both which are healthy to the body. It prevents kidney stone formation.

Things You Need:
Lemons- 3-4
Cold Water- ½ glass
Honey- ¼ tsp

Things You Should Do:
Squeeze the fresh lemons into the cold water.
Mix honey into this solution.
Stir them and drink this juice to cleanse your kidneys from toxins.

Radish Drink for Kidney Cleansing:

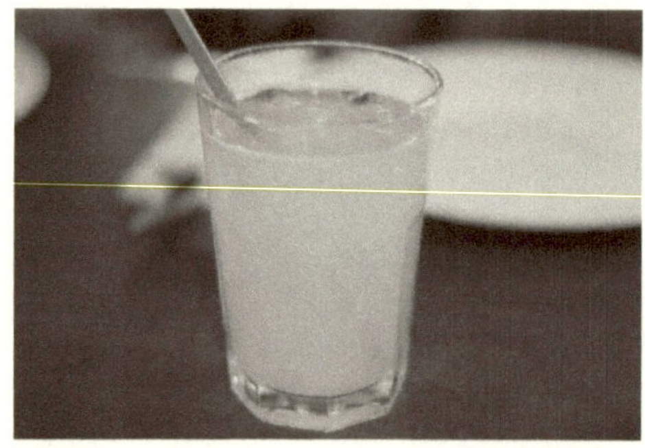

Radishes are great detoxifiers. They work in special regard with the gall bladder and the liver. This will help your kidneys in flushing out the impurities. If you are already a victim of kidney stones, then drinking this radish juice would be one of the best remedies to get rid of your kidney stones. Here is the remedy of radish for kidney cleansing process.

Things You Need:
Radish slices- 1 cup
Purple Cabbage- 1 cup
Celery rib- 1
Things You Should Do:

Wash all the ingredients perfectly.

Get them into a juicer and blend them.

Have this drink to cleanse your kidneys.

Cranberry Juice to cleanse Kidneys:

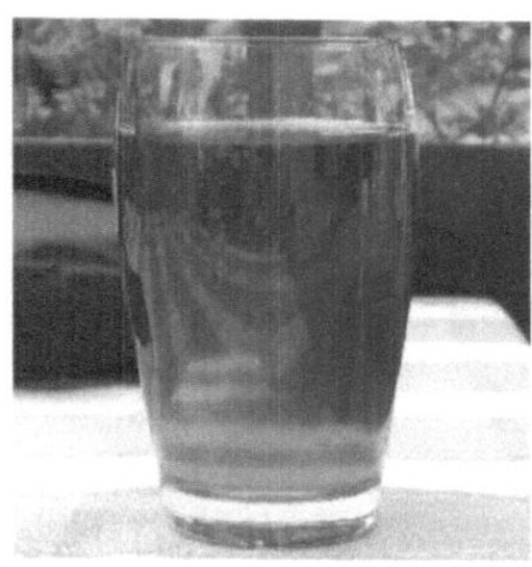

Cranberry juice is another excellent juice that deeply cleans up your kidneys. It is known to be an immensely valued fighter against urinary tract ailments. It also decreases the calcium oxalate content of the kidneys, which is the main cause for the formation of kidney stones. So, use the following recipe to clean up your kidneys.

Things You Need:
    Frozen Cranberries- 500 mg
    Water- 1 liter
    Sugar- 2 tsp
    Cheesecloth- 1

Things You Should Do:
    Wash the cranberries with care.
    Boil the washed cranberries.
    Lessen the flame and cook till the cranberries burst.
    Strain the juice of the cranberries through the cheesecloth.
    Add sugar to upgrade the taste.
    Reheat the juice for a few more minutes.
Have this juice in a chilled form to cleanse your kidneys.

Carrot and Cucumber Juice for Kidney Cleansing:

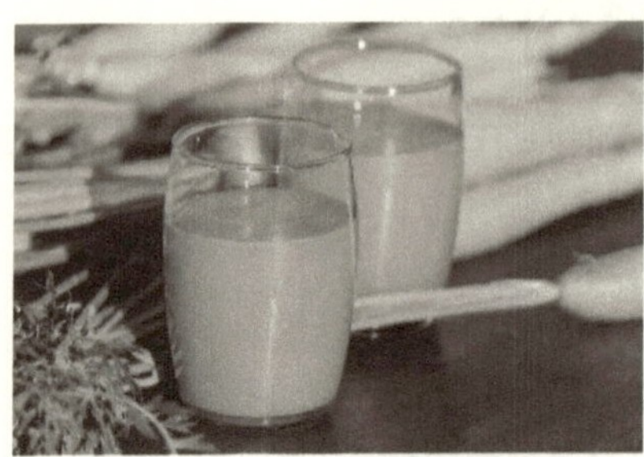

Carrot and cucumber are armed with extensive powers to cleanse kidneys. When combined in a nutritive mix, they tend to flush out all the toxins in a perfect mannerism. Let us see the recipe now:

Things You Need:
Carrots- 2
Cucumber – 1

Things You Should Do:
Chop the carrots and the cucumber into pieces.
Blend them together.
Have this juice regularly to keep your kidneys in an absolved condition.

The herbs to cleanse kidneys work real wonders to clean and tidy up your ever-working kidneys. You might check if you are allergic to any of the herbs before the application of home remedies for the kidneys cleansing process. The herbs do not have any side effects for people without any medical history of allergy.

The details about the herbs and application method is given below: -

Dandelion Root

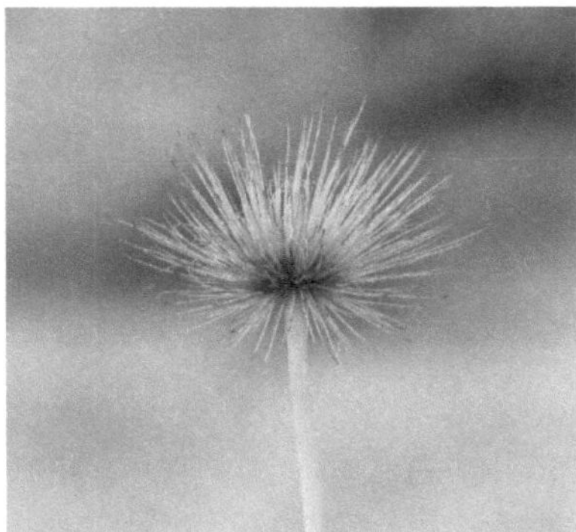

Dandelion works as a great diuretic and promotes the production of more urine. The urination process flush toxins out of the body.

Things You Need:

Dried Dandelion- 1 tsp
Hot water- 1 cup
Honey- ½ tsp

Things You Should Do

Pour the dried dandelion into the hot cup of water.
Allow it to thoroughly get steeped for about 5 minutes of time.
Strain the liquid out and add the honey to it.
Stir the contents together well and sip this tea for about 2 times in a day.

Celery

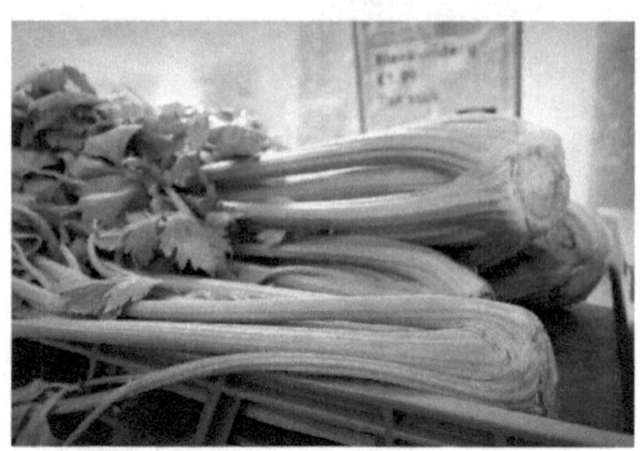

Celery leaves and roots are well known natural diuretic since the ancient times. It comprises of nutrients like potassium and sodium, which makes it the most suitable herb to clean the kidneys.

Things You Need:
Celery Ribs- 2
Fresh Parsley- ½ cup
Cucumber-1
Carrot-1

Things You Should Do:
Blend all the specified ingredients together and prepare a nice juice.
Drink this nutrient-filled juice for about one time in a single day.
Continue doing this for about 2-3 weeks to get best results in cleaning up your kidneys.

Marshmallow

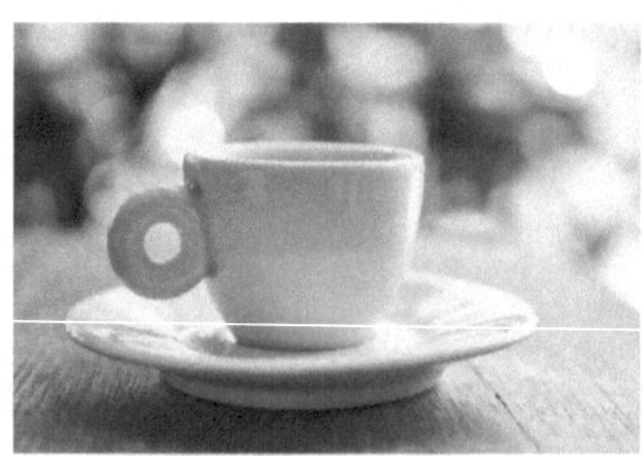

Marshmallows can be effectively used to clean kidneys since they are great diuretics and increases the urine output. This would further improve the health of the kidneys by washing away all kinds of toxins repeatedly.

Things You Need:

Dried Marshmallow root- 1 tbsp.

Hot, boiled water- 1 cup

Things You Should Do:

Add the dried marshmallow root to the hot cup of water.

Allow them to sink for 5-8 minutes and diffuse their flavors out.

Now, strain the liquid out and consume 2 cups of this tea in a single day.

Continue this for up to a week to cleanse your kidneys.

Parsley Drink

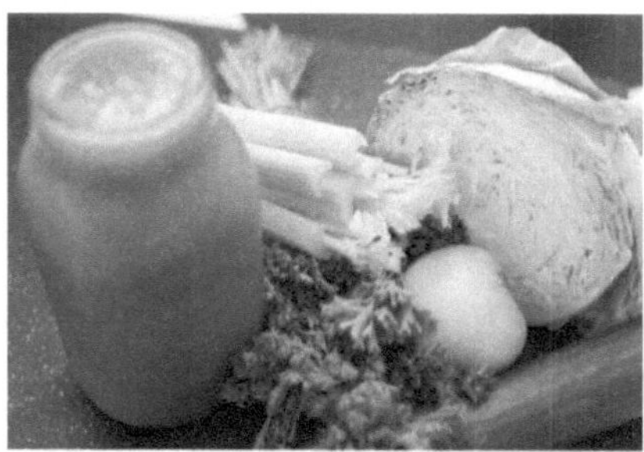

Things You Need:

Parsley Juice- ¼ cup

Water – ½ cup

Honey- ¼ tsp

Lemon juice- ¼ tsp

Things You Should Do:

Mix all the told ingredients together.

Make a fine juice of it.

Drink 2 cups of this juice daily for about 2 weeks to get your kidneys perfectly cleansed.

Ginger

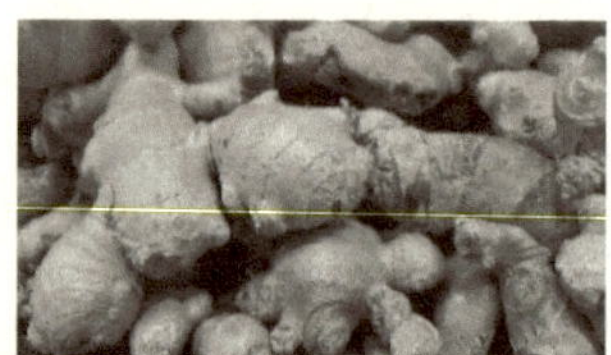

Ginger amazingly improves the process of digestion and also wash off harmful microbial content of the body. This is a great herb which you can use to perfectly conduct kidney cleansing process.

Things You Need:

Grated Ginger- 2 tsp

Hot boiled water- 2 cups

Honey- ½ tsp

Lemon Juice- ¼ tsp

Things You Should Do:

Add the grated ginger to the hot water.

Allow them to steep together for about at least 4-9 minutes.

Add the lemon juice and the honey to it and stir them all well.

Have 2 cups of this tea daily.

Repeat the same for about a few weeks to get your kidneys cleansed.

Horsetail

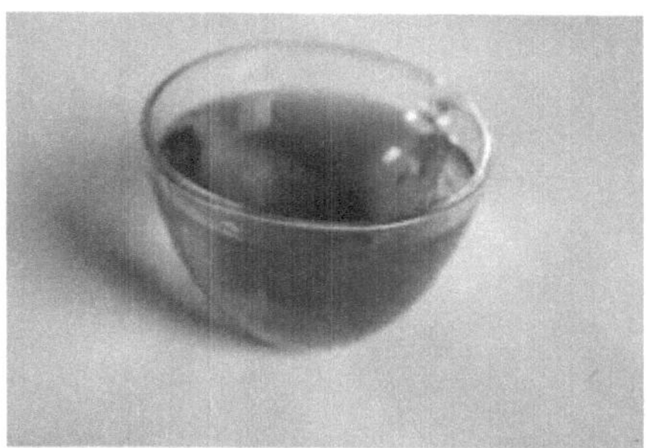

Horsetail is yet another wonderful and a striking herb that can lead to an entire cleaning of your kidneys astoundingly. This is also a natural diuretic and can be very much helpful to clean the kidneys. Also, it is an excellent antioxidant which provides an immense help in intensely cleaning the renal system.

Things You Need:
 Dried horsetail- 1-3 tsp
 Hot water- 1 cup
Things You Should Do:
 Add the dried horsetail to the hot boiling water.
 Allow it to mix thoroughly by waiting for about 7-8 minutes.
 Now, strain the liquid out and sip on 2 cups of this tea in a day.
 Continue to do this for about 1 week to clean your kidneys.

Other Tips to Sufficiently Cleanse your Kidneys at home:

Apart from what all has been mentioned above, here are a few handful tips which would serve you the best in cleaning your kidneys.

Drink a lot of water is one of the basic tip which you should follow to keep your kidneys clean. Water acts as a great solvent and would aid you in flushing out all the harmful and unneeded toxins from your body.

Cleansing can also be rightly done when you introduce the practice of drinking various juices and healthy liquid combinations. These can include fruit juices, vegetable juices or a combination of both.

Try to avoid smoking and high consumption of alcohol as it is very harmful for your kidneys.

Keep a close eye on your cholesterol levels and if you are an overweight person, try to reduce your weight considerably.

Avert yourself away from foods that are processed and fried.

Keep yourself inclined to food which is healthy. Examples are leafy vegetables, whole grain foods, fresh fruits, etc.

Work hard to keep your blood sugar levels and blood pressure levels in check.

Exercise regularly.

Liver Detox

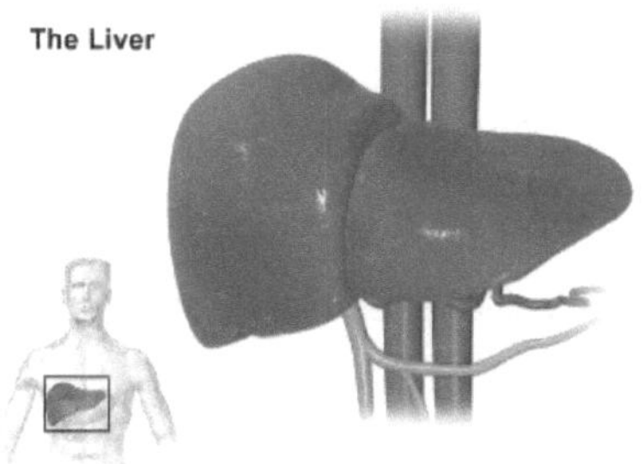

Ten signs your liver is telling you, it needs help

abdominal bloating

pain or discomfort over the liver – (right upper abdominal area under the rib cage)

excessive abdominal fat; pot belly; or a roll around the upper abdomen

trouble in digestion

pain in gallbladder

acid reflux/heartburn

dark spots on the skin commonly referred to liver spots

overheating of the body & excessive perspiration

weight gain and inability to lose weight even with calorie restriction

Worst Foods for Your Liver

Animal-Based Foods

A damaged liver is unable to metabolize proteins properly and break down the amino acids produced in the body from eating animal-based foods. Avoid red meat, such as beef and bison. As well, you should eliminate or limit the eggs and dairy products you eat. Dairy may include milk, cheese and yogurt. Protein is important in overall nutrition, so opt for lean meats from poultry and non-meat protein sources such as beans and nuts. You may also consider trying plant-based products such as soy milk.

High-Sodium Foods

Salt contains sodium, which is not processed completely by a damaged liver. Canned foods, including soups, meats or vegetables, are high in salt and sugar, which cause abdominal swelling and fluid retention. Following a low-sodium diet is optimal for preventing further liver damage as well as unnecessary inflammation. Use garlic, pepper or spices to flavor foods instead of salt.

Sugary Foods

Avoid sugary foods such as candy, ice cream and cake and salty foods like potato chips, which are simple carbohydrates with high levels of sugar and sodium, respectively. Eat foods with natural sugars and fibrous carbs, such as strawberries, oranges or apples, to avoid unhealthy levels of sugar and sodium in your liver.

Alcohol

Depending on the severity of damage to your liver, a chance for regeneration can occur if you abstain from all alcoholic beverages. Chronic alcoholism contributes to the onset of liver damage because it inhibits proper absorption of nutrients, forcing the liver to become toxic. Avoid drinking beer, wine or champagne as well as any form of liquor. Take note that some over-the-counter pain medications also contain alcohol, such as cough syrup.

Fried Foods

We all know fried foods, particularly those from fast food restaurants, have a negative effect on our liver, but it turns out eating French fries, extra crispy chicken or deep-fried cheese-filled wontons influence our liver that's very similar to hepatitis. Eating fried foods has also been shown to elevate bad cholesterol and lower good cholesterol.

Trans Fats

Trans fat-loaded foods, or foods containing partially hydrogenated oils, are far from a thing of the past, still showing up in processed foods everywhere, like store-bought frosting, salad dressing, microwave popcorn, crackers, cookies. Even small amounts of trans fats increase bad cholesterol...fast! In fact, all the extra LDLs from trans fats get dumped into our liver, increasing the risk of disease.

Large doses of iron

Taking more iron supplements than recommended can cause serious liver damage. This is because the body has no way of eliminating excess iron, so it accumulates in the organs and tissues, including the liver. Too much iron can cause liver scarring which in some cases can lead to cirrhosis, a condition where the liver slowly deteriorates and malfunctions. Excess iron can also increase a person's risk of developing liver cancer.

Cigarettes

If you smoke cigarettes there's a chance that you are causing damage to your liver – increasing your risk of developing liver cancer and decreasing your liver's ability to rid your body of dangerous toxins. In turn, this could leave you more susceptible to the damaging effects of some medications on the liver too.

Some over-the-counter medications

Even over-the-counter medications should be taken with caution – always follow the directions on the packaging. Paracetamol for example, when taken in excessive amounts can be very toxic to the liver, especially when taken together with alcohol. If you already have liver disease, aspirin should be taken with care. Non-steroidal anti-inflammatory drugs like Advil (ibuprofen) and diclofenac can also be dangerous for people with liver disease.

Foods and herbs that may keep the liver clean

These are the list of food that keeps your liver clean

Dandelion Root , Avocado, Lemon juice, Turmeric, Garlic, Water, Brussels Sprouts, Fasting, Coffee ,Enemas, Bananas, Coffee Enemas, Sweet potatoes, Tomato sauce, Blackstrap Molasses ,Beans, Beet Greens and Spinach

Detox drinks to cleanse Liver

Dandelion Root

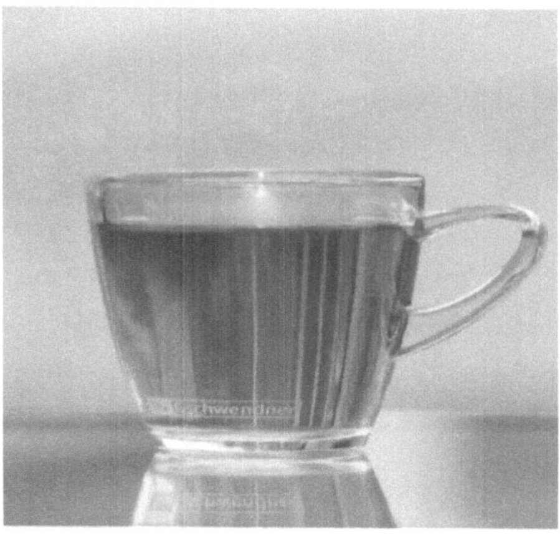

Dandelion root has amazing healing powers. It has been used for eons as a healing liver tincture—steeped as a tea or brewed as a bitter coffee. Many Korean and Mexican forms of herbal medicine utilize dandelion for its powerful antioxidant hepatoprotective properties.

dandelion root had therapeutic properties as it has the kynurenic acid within. This amino acid is used for digestive aid support, specifically for bile production, and luckily dandelion root has the richest concentration needed to stimulate bile production and bile transport toxins out of the body. Therefore, dandelion root is considered a strong natural liver detoxifying agent.

Avocados

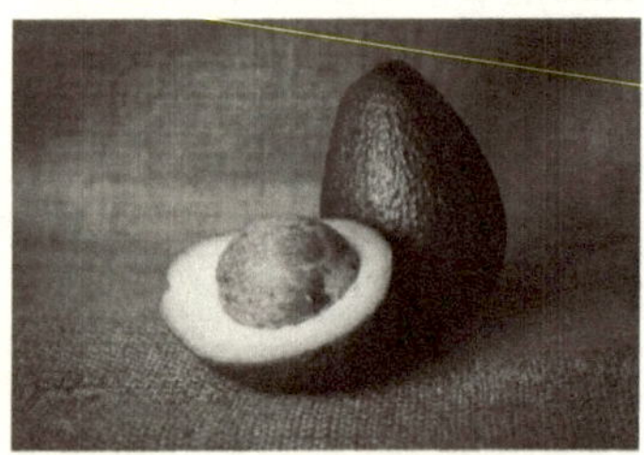

It turns out that in addition to be a great source of healthy fats, the yummy, creamy avocado is great for your liver. In fact, a Japanese study discovered that avocados packed with protective compounds that shield the liver from damaging toxins, like galactosa mine. These compounds, in which avocados are rich, help protect the liver from long term damage. Avocados happen to by high in glutathione, a powerful antioxidant that can repair damaged cells in your liver.

Lemon / Lime

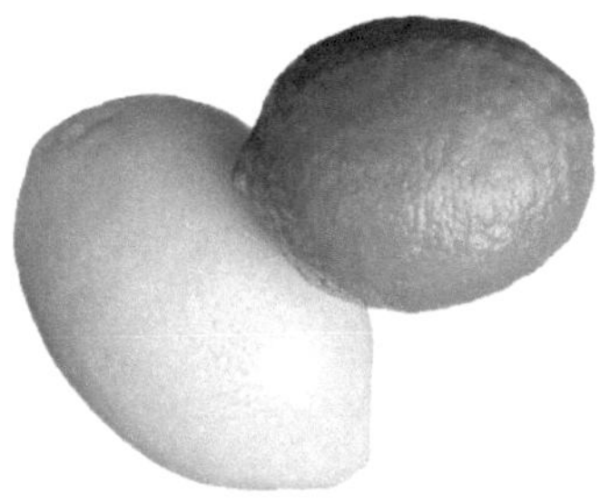

Lemon has naturally cleansing abilities. Just look in your kitchen to see just how many cleaning products have lemon as an ingredient. In fact, if you use green or DIY safe cleaners, you don't need much more than lemon to give your kitchen a clean, lively, refreshing smell. Well, the same things go for the inside of your body.

Turmeric

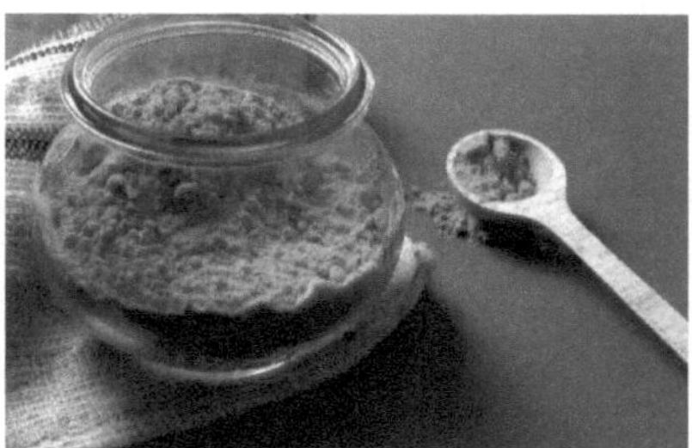

If you suffer from chronic inflammation or liver issues, turmeric is a potent spice with serious anti-inflammatory benefits. Turmeric has proven effective in warding off nasty viral infections. Turmeric has long been used in naturally healing for its beneficial effects on our bodies and organs.

It just so happens that turmeric spice is rich in curcumin, an active pharmacological agent with powerful anti-bacterial, antiseptic, antiviral, anti-fungal, anti-carcinogenic, and anti-inflammatory abilities. With a blast of inner body benefits, this spice is a superhero protecting our livers from evil infections and damage, and giving liver cells the boost they need to regenerate fresh, healthy tissues.

Adding it to our diet regularly also helps to increase our levels of natural bile production – essential to ridding our bodies of harmful toxins.

Garlic

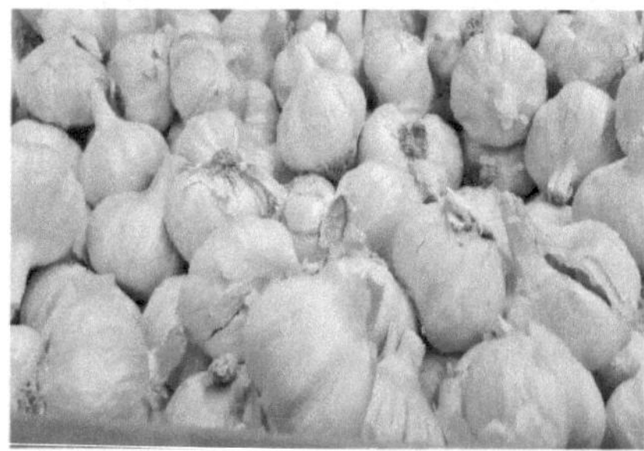

In addition to its supernatural expertise in warding off vampires, a small clove of garlic is anti-viral. Not only does garlic help beef up the immune system to ward of infections and germs, garlic packs pungent sulfur compounds, which trigger the function of enzymes to enhance liver function. This is due to the high levels of sulfur compounds in garlic. These can encourage enzyme production in the liver.

If that wasn't already beneficial enough, garlic is high in source of selenium and allicin, both agents that act to protect our livers. And luckily, the taste and versatility of garlic means it's super easy to incorporate into daily diets for a healthier, protected, and detoxed liver.

Water

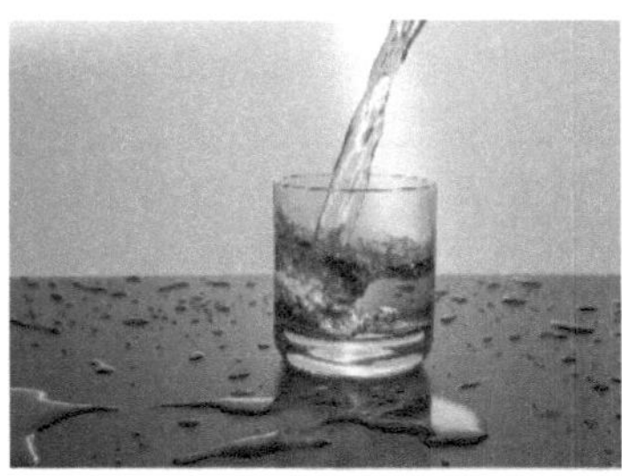

Drinking water all by itself is a way to help flush the body of toxins daily, but with a few simple ingredients you can transform water into a detoxifying masterpiece and reap even more benefits from it. This is something you can do every single day, or as part of a broader detoxing program. Herbal tea and water infused with lemon, improve waste elimination and protect the liver from developing gallstones. You already know that your liver primarily works to filter the blood that is transported from your digestive tract, to metabolize nutrients, as well as to filter out drugs, alcohol, and other toxins. Each one of the ingredients listed here will provide slightly different benefits, so be sure to choose it according to the goal you have.

Brussels Sprouts

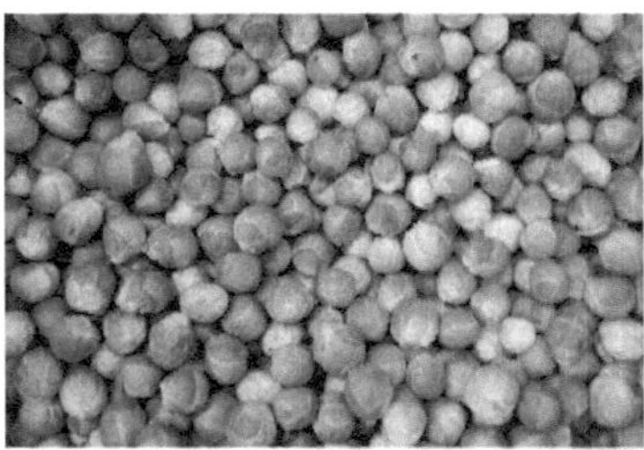

They might taste a little funky, but Brussels sprouts contain glucosinolate, a Sulphur compound that gives off that telltale pungent smell while shielding the liver from toxic and chemical damage. So, invite a few more of these "mini-cabbages" to you next diner party. According to the National Cancer Institute, cruciferous vegetables contain glucosinolate, a collection of substances that contain sulfur chemicals, which is why Brussels sprouts have such a pungent aroma and bitter flavor.

However, Brussels sprouts also contain glucosinolates, which help form biologically active compounds (i.e., nitriles, indoles, isothiocyanates and thiocyanates) that are credited by the National Cancer Institute, as well as other noted medical experts, for their anticancer effects on the liver and other essential organs.

Fasting

Fasting is an ancient religious practice that may have some surprising benefits for modern health. While the scientific community is far from a consensus, there is evidence that suggests fasting stimulates a surprising array of positive influences on the body. While there are known risks involved with fasting that need to be accounted for, unexpected benefits are coming into clearer focus as well.

Fasting influences everything from the immune system to mental health to weight loss. This may indicate that our obsession with what we eat has been misplaced. Instead, perhaps our focus should be on when we eat. Here are eight things you should know about fasting...

Here are how fasting benefits your health in a nutshell. Fasting puts a mild stress on the body that stimulates a positive response, sort of like exercising a muscle. You need to put stress on it via exercise for it to grow stronger. Except in this case, depriving your system of calories puts stress on your entire body so there is a more broad-based effect

With your immune system, hunger triggers a recycling process that reduces the amount of damaged or unused immune cells to save energy. This helps fight against many common autoimmune problems like arthritis, lupus, and type 1 diabetes. With detoxification, fasting helps expunge the toxins stored in your fat cells. Additionally, after a few days, fasting also leads to a higher production of endorphins in the bloodstream leading to a more positive sense of wellbeing. Finally, reducing caloric intake reduces stress on your internal organs and can help them go the extra mile later in life in effect prolonging your lifespan.

Sweet Potatoes

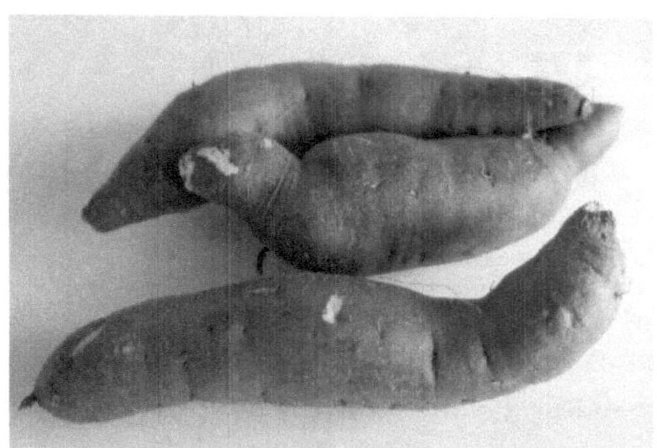

Surprisingly, it is not the banana that is the richest in potassium. It is the sweet potato. A single medium sweet potato contains nearly 700 milligrams of potassium, not to mention the high fiber and beta-carotene content.

A sweet potato only has 131 calories, yet is rich with Vitamins B-6, C, D, magnesium and iron. While naturally sweet, the sugars are slowly released into the bloodstream through the liver, without causing a spike in blood sugar.

Beet Greens and Spinach

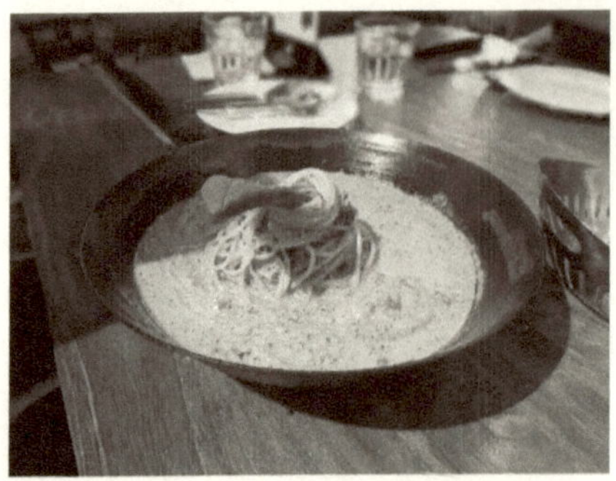

Rich in anti-oxidants, beet greens contain over 1300 milligrams of potassium per cup. Add beets and beet greens to your fresh vegetable juice recipe, finely chop and add raw to salads, or sauté lightly, like other greens. Beets also naturally cleanse the gallbladder and improve bile flow. Fresh organic spinach is easily added to your diet, and is a good source of potassium, containing 840 milligrams per serving.

Beans

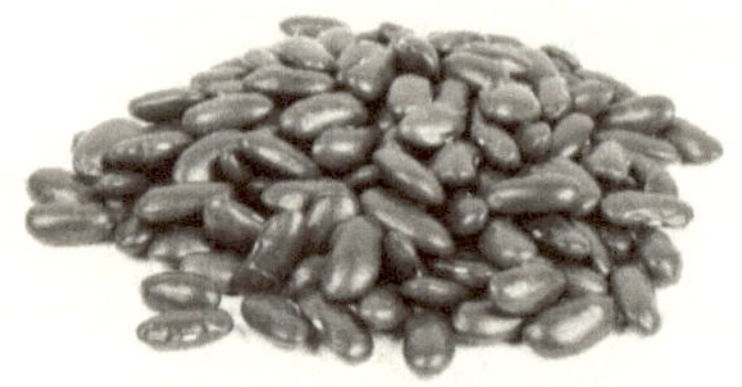

White beans, kidney beans and lima beans are all rich with potassium, protein and fiber. Swap out one of these potassium rich beans for garbanzo beans in your favorite hummus recipe and eat with carrot sticks and celery sticks.

Bananas

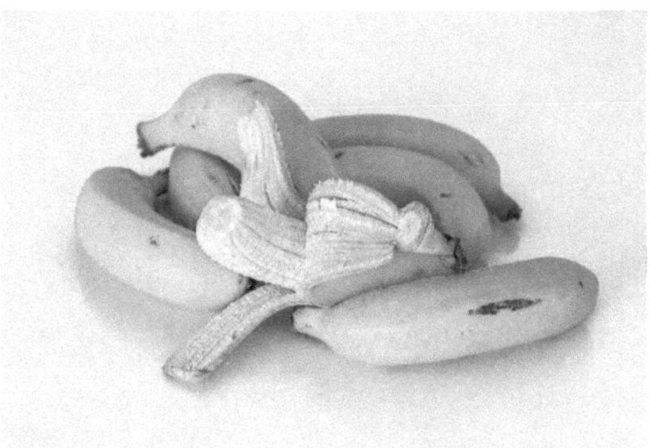

And finally, add a banana to your favorite smoothie. While in comparison to the other high potassium foods on this list, the banana's 470 milligrams of potassium are only part of the story. Bananas assist in digestion and help to release toxins and heavy metals from the body – all of which are essential during a liver cleanse.

Heart Detox

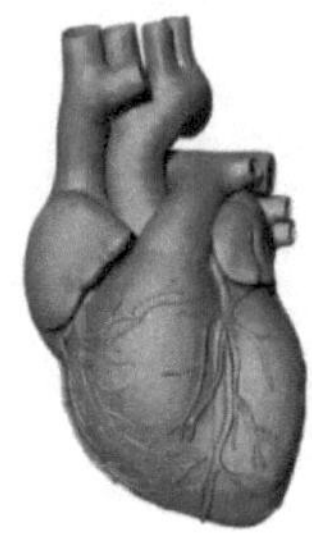

Ten signs your heart is telling you, it needs help

Swollen, Bleeding, Sore Gums

Snoring and Sleep Apnea

Swollen Feet and Legs

Coughing

Dizziness

Fatigue

No appetite and Nausea

Sweating

Weakness

<u>Foods to cleanse your arteries</u>

Foods can effectively remove blockages in the arteries and maintain a healthy heart. Here are 20 best heart healthy foods to cleanse your arteries.

Orange

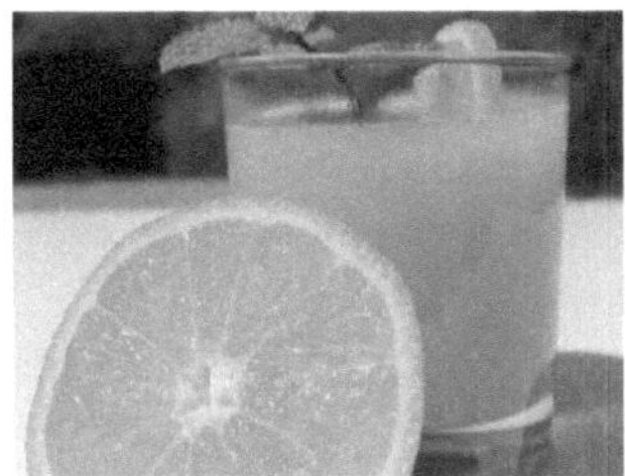

Orange is a powerhouse of vitamin C that can fight common cold. But this fruit can also fight heart diseases, here's how. Oranges contain fiber pectin that lowers cholesterol; vitamin C strengthens the walls of the artery and sweeps out blockages. Orange juice can improve the functioning of the blood vessels.

Pomegranate

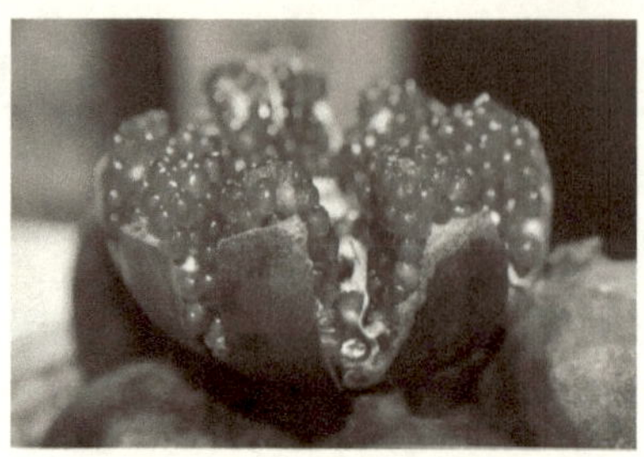

Fruits rich with antioxidants improve the walls of the arteries. Pomegranate is especially heart-friendly due to the presence of phytochemicals that are an antioxidant. Pomegranate ignites the production of nitric oxide that improves the flow of blood and expands the arteries.

Broccoli

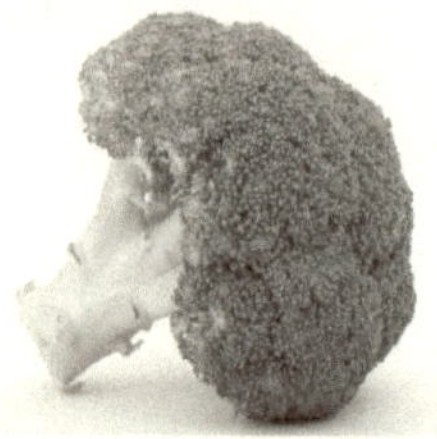

Broccoli is a good source for proteins for vegetarians. Broccoli contains vitamin K which is beneficial for bone formation. Vitamin K also protects the arteries from damage. Besides vitamin K, broccoli is rich in fiber, which can lower cholesterol and high blood pressure.

Whole grain

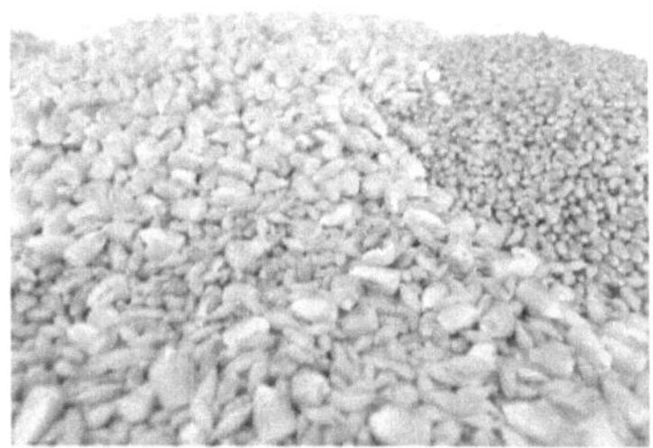

Whole Wheat, Whole Oats, Brown Rice, Whole Rye, Freekeh, Whole-Grain Barley, Buckwheat, Bulgur are most popular whole grains which should be included in your daily diet to reduce cholesterol. Whole grains contain fibers that push out the blockages.

Fatty fish

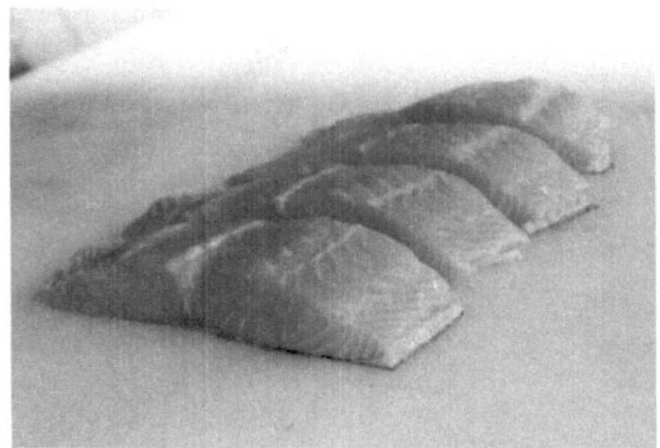

Seafood is beneficial on various levels – Mental health, brain, vision, building muscles and pregnancy. The truth is that Omega 3 fatty acids are the remedies for these problems. Omega 3 can also protect your heart and reduce blood triglyceride levels.

Nuts

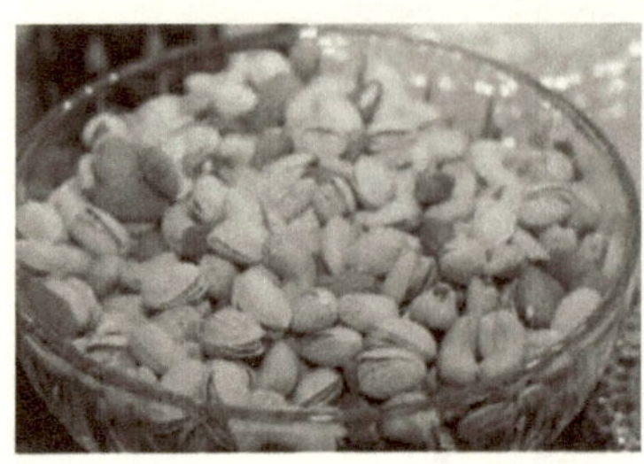

Almonds, peanuts, walnuts or hazelnuts are heart-friendly nuts. These nuts contain vitamin E that can protect the walls of the arteries. Nuts also contain fibers that also help to reduce cholesterol in the blood.

Olive oil

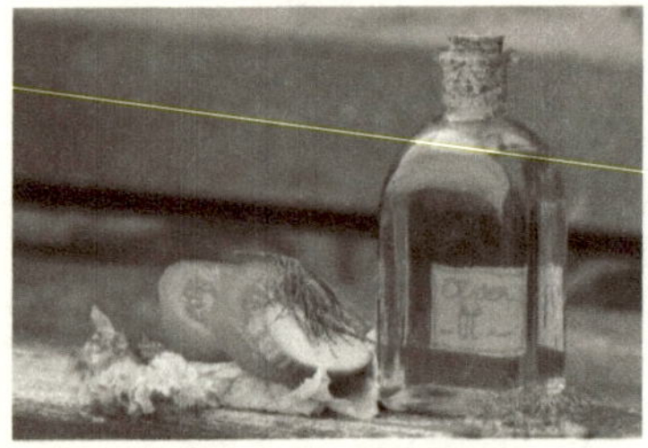

Olive oil is known to have several health benefits, but it is the best oil to prevent a build-up of cholesterol in the blood. Besides cholesterol, olive oil can also reduce high blood pressure. Olive oil comes under monounsaturated and polyunsaturated fats, which are both beneficial fats for the body.

Cinnamon

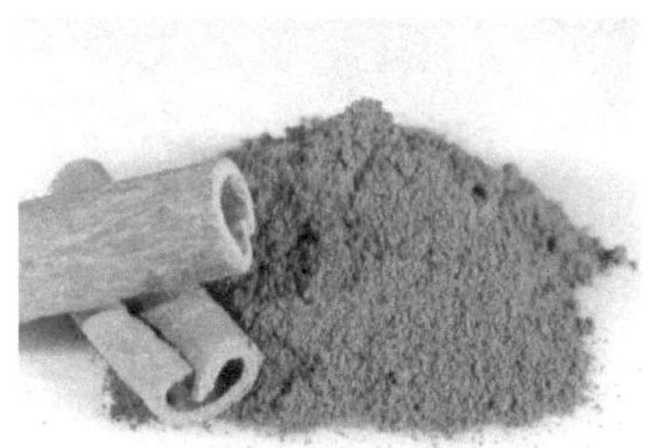

This spice should be brought in the limelight for the several health benefits it caters to overall health. Cinnamon is used as a spice as well as for dessert. This versatile spice lowers fat in the blood preventing blockages in the vessels.

Tea

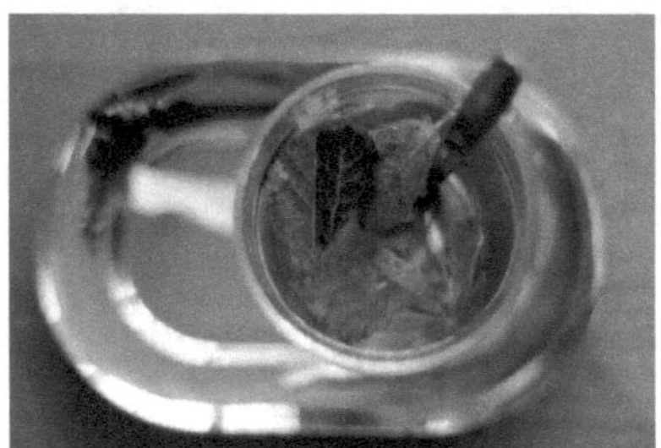

Tea can increase your metabolism for weight, but it can also improve heart health. Tea contains an antioxidant called catechins that acts like a shield to the artery wall. These antioxidants also prevent blood clots that can be fatal.

Watermelon

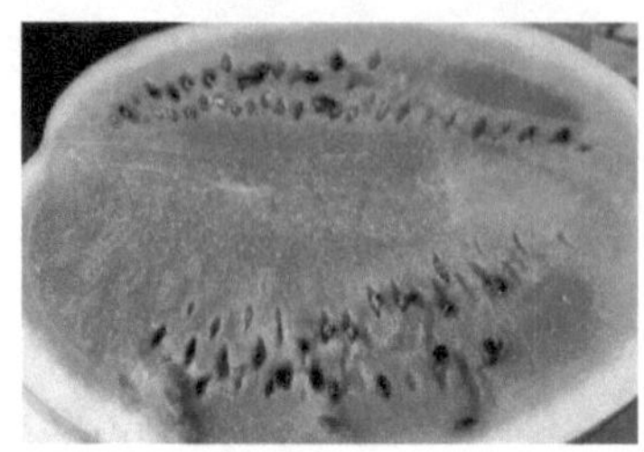

Watermelon works great for skin care treatment, as a detox and a weight loss food. Amino acid found in watermelon helps reduce high blood pressure. But watermelon also contains nitric oxide which opens the blood vessels to improve the flow of blood.

Spinach

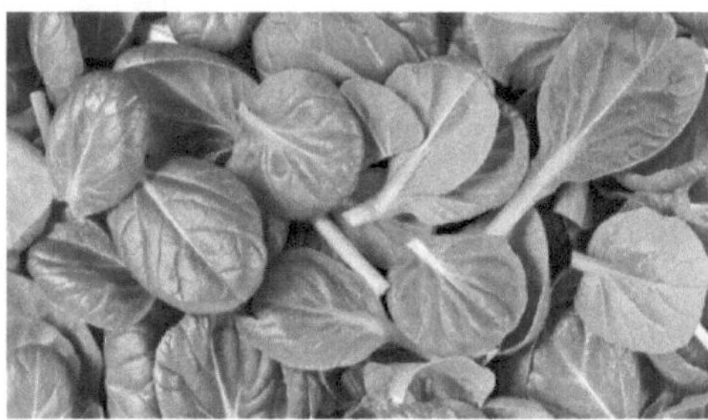

Spinach is another fierce ingredient to fight heart diseases. Spinach contains carotene that prevents cholesterol from getting clogged in the arteries. Spinach can reduce high blood pressure to due to the nutrients and minerals present in it.

Tomato

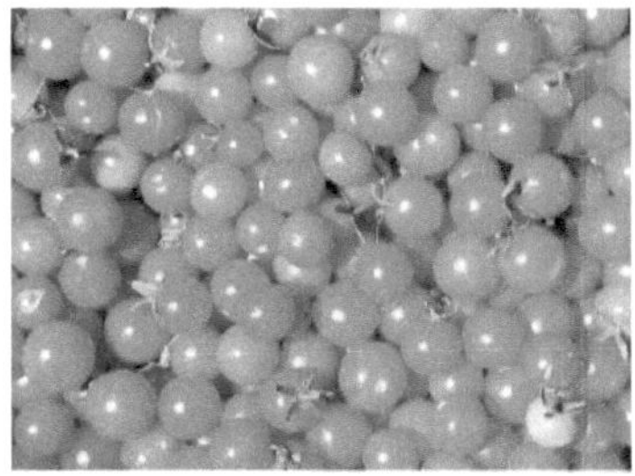

Like pomegranate and tea, tomato too contains antioxidants that protects the arterial walls. In tomatoes, lycopene keeps the cholesterol levels low. If the tomato sauce for your pizza is prepared from fresh ingredients, then it is a healthy pizza.

Beans

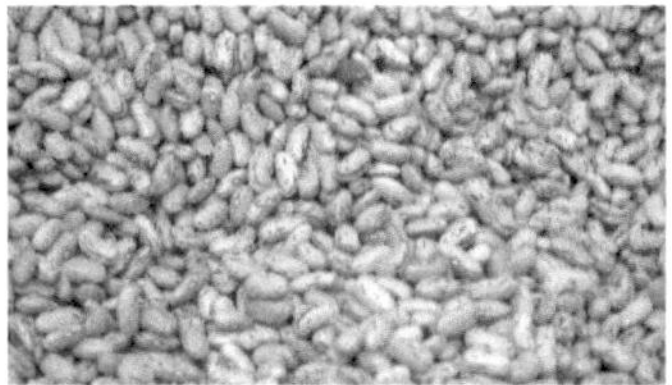

Beans contain fiber and folic acid that prevents arteries from getting clogged. Beans are also a good source of carbohydrates and plant proteins.

Apples

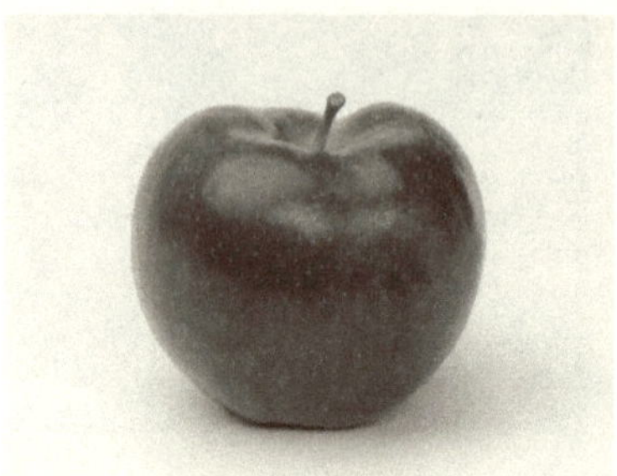

Like oranges, apples too contain a fiber called pectin that absorbs cholesterol from the blood. Apples are a great way to reduce cholesterol as you can have it anytime, anywhere and you consume it the way you want. Slice them or have it as a dessert, apple is an all-time favorite to improve health.

Grapefruit

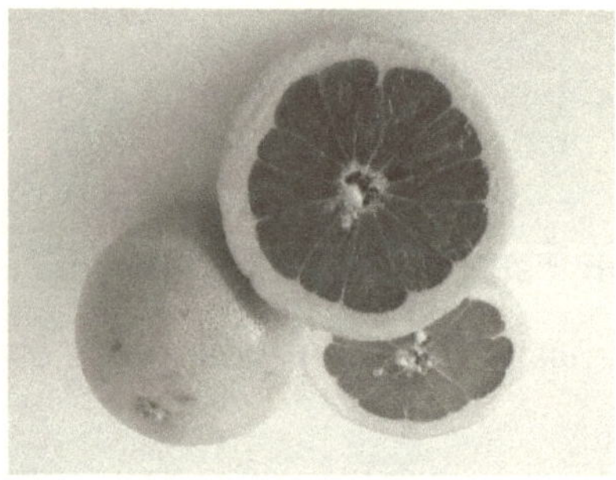

The pink grapefruit is rich in antioxidant, lycopene which is also present in tomatoes. Pink grapefruit helps prevent damage to your arteries. Grapefruit is also a great fruit for diabetics.

Corn

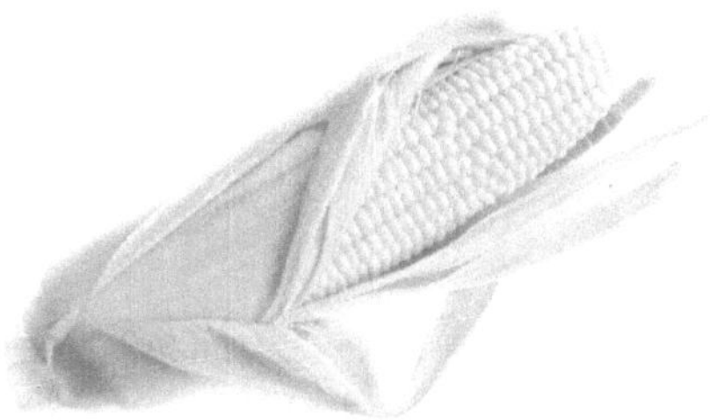

Protect your arteries by consuming corn or maize. Corn contains fiber that protects your arteries by flushing out cholesterol.

Turmeric

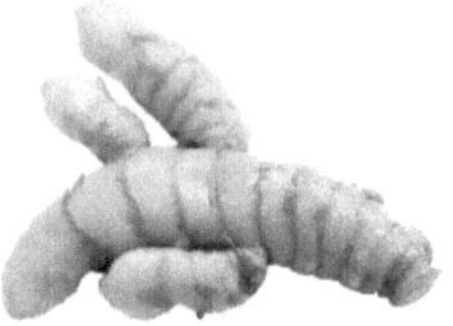

Turmeric has anti-inflammatory properties. This spice works in favor of reducing heart diseases. Curcumin that's present in turmeric reduces inflammation in the arteries and the deposits of fats or blockages.

Colon Detox

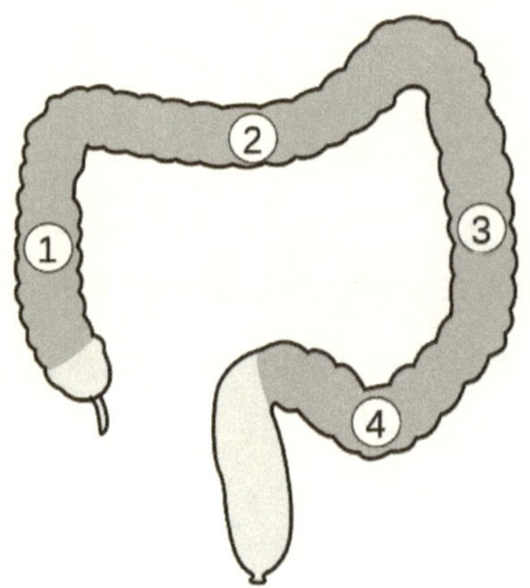

<u>Worst Foods for Your Colon</u>

High-fat and fried food

Chili peppers

Dairy

Alcohol

Chocolate

Coffee, tea, and soft drinks

Corn

Refine flour

Foods to cleanse your Colon

Apple

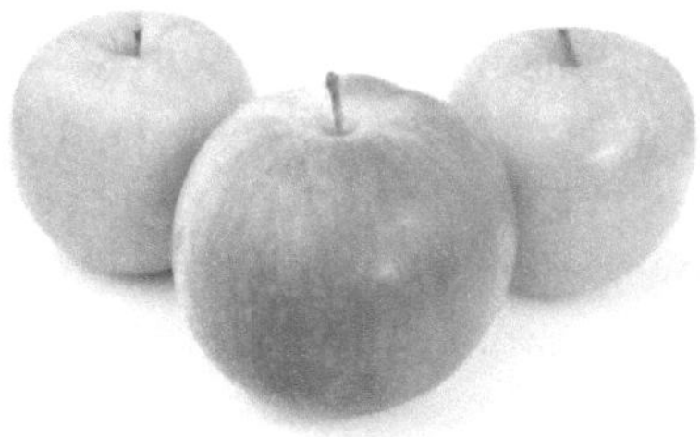

Many advanced colon-cleansing protocols include either whole apples, apple sauce, apple juice, or apple cider vinegar (ACV) because this simple fruit is a powerful cleansing food. High in fiber, a nutrient that is already widely known to promote healthy digestion, apples are also rich in pectin, a carbohydrate compound that acts as a thickening agent inside the gut. When taken in therapeutic doses, pectin can help root out built-up toxins in the colon and strengthen the intestinal lining.

Avocados

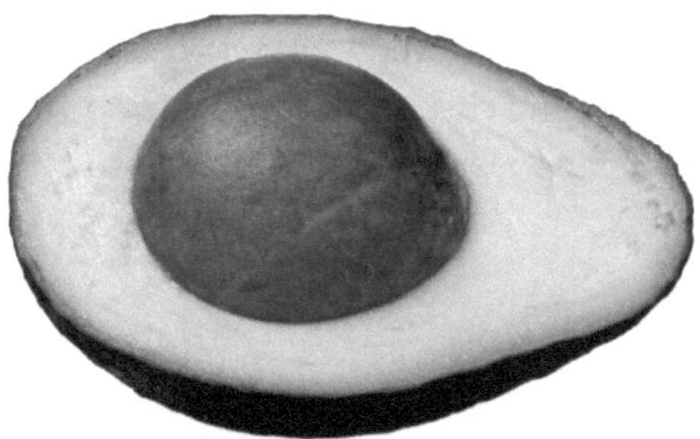

For everyday colon cleansing, avocados are another great option for detoxification and digestion. Like apples, avocados are rich in fiber, and include both soluble and insoluble varieties at a ratio of about one to three, which is quite unique. And as it turns out, insoluble fiber is the type that promotes healthy bowel movements and cleanses the colon effectively reducing one's overall risk of developing colon cancer.

Also important is the avocado's soluble fiber content, which is important for absorbing water and binding with other digested substances to help them easily move through the digestive tract. This mechanistic "gelling" effect also helps maintain bowel regularity in its own unique way and prevents the toxic buildups that can lead to irregularity and constipation.

Flax and chia seeds

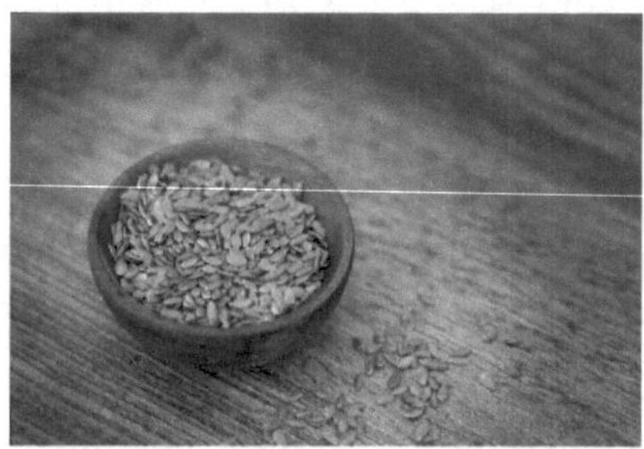

Unique in their nutritional profiles, both flax and chia seeds possess fats and fiber that help promote healthy digestion and a clean colon. Both are rich in omega-3 fatty acids, for instance, which have been shown to stabilize cell walls and reduce inflammation. Flax and chia also contain their own unique blends of soluble fiber, which bind with food to optimize the digestive process.

Chlorophyll-rich greens

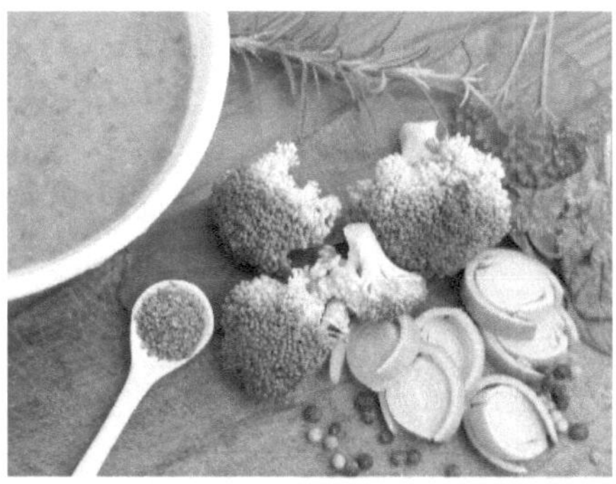

Green fruits and vegetables that are rich in chlorophyll tend to promote healthy digestion and daily colon cleaning as well. Spinach, green olives, asparagus, Brussels sprouts, cabbage, celery, collard greens, sea vegetables, leeks, peas, and Swiss chard are all high in chlorophyll, which means they can help cleanse your digestive tract and detoxify your liver. Supplementing with liquid chlorophyll is another option for boosting intake of this important nutrient for maximum colon health.

"Fat-soluble chlorophyll adheres to the lining of the intestinal wall and retards bacterial growth, removes putrefactive bacteria from the colon, and helps heal the mucosal lining of the gastrointestinal tract.

Clean water with sea salt

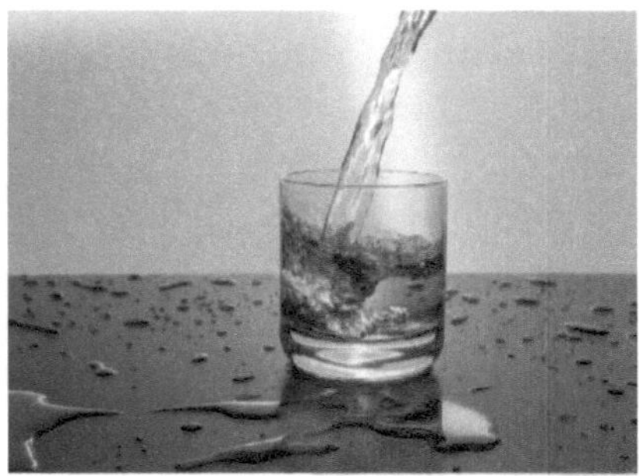

A hydrated colon is a healthy colon. Perpetual dehydration can lead to constipation and toxic buildup, which is why it is important to drink plenty of clean, fluoride-free water every day. Some experts recommend drinking at least half your body weight in ounces of water every single day for maximum hydration and cleansing. You can also add some sea salt to your water to help further promote detoxification.

Fermented foods

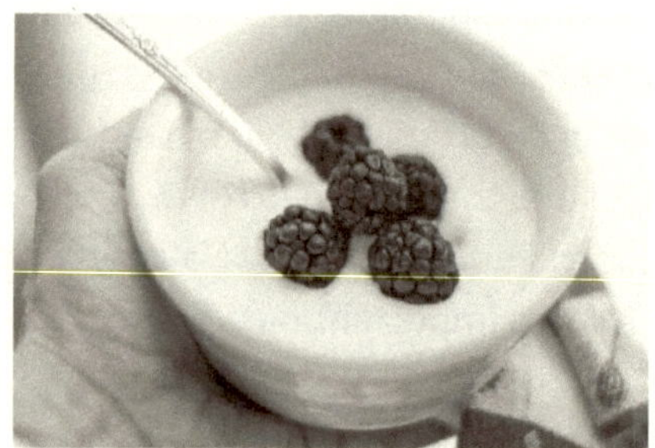

The human digestive system is composed of a vast network of beneficial microbiota that are responsible for digesting food, absorbing nutrients, thwarting harmful bacteria, and eliminating toxins. When these bacteria get thrown out of balance, however, digestive health can suffer -- and the longer this bacterial balance is out of whack, the more severe the damage that can ensue.

To help offset the damage to your gut flora caused by environmental and food chemicals, antibiotic drugs, processed foods, and other factors, it is important to supplement with probiotic bacteria and eat plenty of fermented, probiotic-rich foods. These include cultured vegetables like kimchi, and fermented beverages like kombucha tea and kefir.

Check out our other bestselling books :

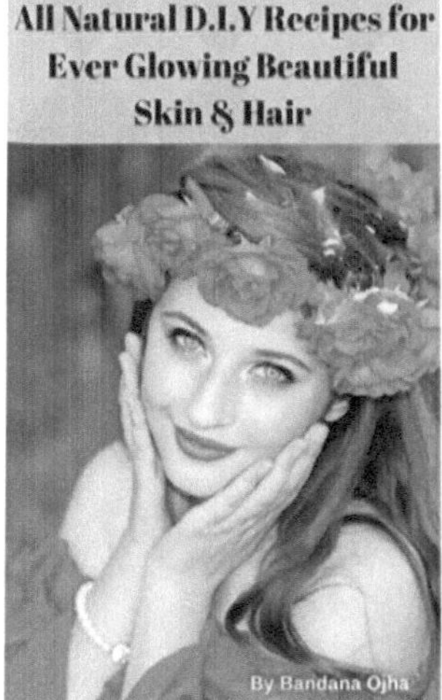

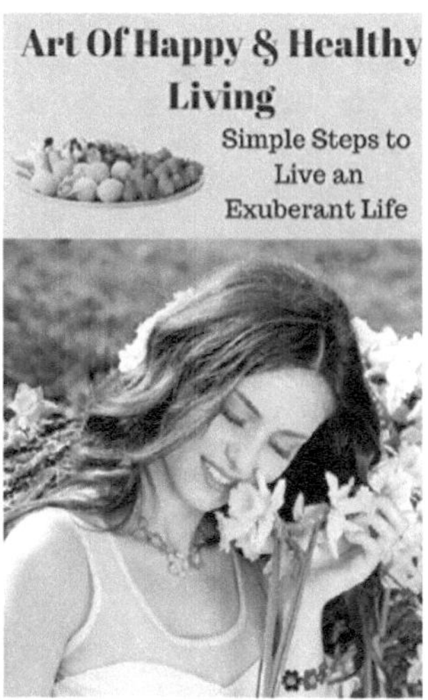